CHRIST HEALED ME

Even in the terminal stage of an illness Christ can perform a miracle Based on real facts.

From
Kenia Adit Acevedo Martínez
☐

© Copyright 2020. Kenia Adit Acevedo Martínez. All rights reserved.
It is illegal to reproduce, copy or distribute any part of this document in digital or paper format. Registration of this publication is strictly prohibited.

Dedication

This book is dedicated to:
God, my beloved Heavenly Father who, with immeasurable displays of love every day when we wake up, reminds me that he never leaves us alone, his grace surrounds us.

Introduction

In daily life, many times we are limited in our way of perceiving things, we often visit places, we meet people, but, there is very little information that we can appreciate and receive in our memory, because we are continuously agitated thinking about our commitments, be it work, studies or simply the routine to which we have immersed ourselves.

We are aware of what is happening around, but not precisely focused on what really matters.

We often have distractions such as fashions, entertainment and an endless number of things that often do nothing to benefit our existence, we lose sight of the family, nature and most importantly of our lives God is many times distant because of the enormous wall that we build of occupations and distractions that mostly capture our attention and separate us from it.

But when we are in circumstances that completely compromise our being, which exceed our human capacity to resolve it, it is until then when we look up to the sky in search of answers, in search of solution, in search of help.

In this book we are going to find something that surpasses what is humanly possible and as incredible as it may seem, it is part of the reality between us "The Divine Healing", it goes beyond the human because, as the term divine correctly says, it only comes from God , our sovereign creator, our eternal King and Heavenly Father who lives forever, who loves us in such a way that he gave his only son Jesus Christ so that all who believe in him will not perish but have eternal life, as quoted in the Bible in the book of Saint John chapter 3 verse 16, God's unequaled love for humanity is palpable as you are right now reading these lines.

I hope dear reader that through this book you can open your attention so that Christ himself speaks to your life and deals with your heart, just as he did with me.

Chapter One: In the transit of life

Each day that begins brings with it challenges and hopes for a better future, but such are often unnoticed due to this routine in daily life.

We are used to doing the same things, visiting the same places, the same people, and that's fine, but when something comes into our lives that is totally contrary to our routine, our world seems to wobble and spin out of control.

In this chapter I want to tell you that perhaps we are not that different in our way of living. Normally I used to wake up early in the morning, look for something to eat healthy as indicated by the advice of the daily live on social networks or in the tips of your favorite nutrition magazine; We tried to live a healthy and remarkably normal life, I was no exception, I tried to eat a well-proportioned diet, a peacefully balanced rhythm of life, I did my exercise time in the gym in the morning.

I was doing the final stage of my university studies, everything seemed to be going great because for a young person full of health, with an adequate pace of life, about to finish their university studies, with new goals to carry out and generally always happy visiting the room from time to time.

It could be said that it was everything that a young woman today does normally and everything happened relatively normally in this cycle, I remind myself that at the time when I was almost finishing my university studies something very special happened, I had the opportunity to Visiting an evangelical Christian church and listening to the message of love and salvation that Christ gives, but he still could not understand the magnitude of what his love meant, he heard it, but he did not understand it.

Even so, when I heard that someone was able to give himself like this just for love, I could feel in my heart as if that something that I had not yet managed to achieve in my life, that unknown something that nothing filled, neither diets, nor exercises, nor academic achievement, nothing filled a space inside me that without understanding it seemed to have found its exact complement at that time, Christ was the answer that my heart needed but I did not accept it, perhaps due to the harshness of the past, situations that unintentionally leave internal traces that it is difficult for us to recognize and therefore it is difficult to heal them, since the first step to heal a wound, is to recognize that you exist and that you need help.

Although I felt all this within me, no change came about in my life that day, because I did not allow my heart to open up and let Christ restore it.

Chapter Two: No matches

I came home and as I tuned in to my favorite secular music radio, something happened.

The radio that I had and that generally due to some defect I think, or I'm not sure if there was a purpose in it, generally changed the station every time the power went out or some similar situation happened.

I had to turn on the radio again, but he lost his tune, he did not continue with the station he had on, so while trying to find the secular music radio that he had been listening to, he passed by another without realizing it and stopped a bit time to listen to what the person singing was saying.

He said that although he came from a life wrapped in drugs, the hard life of the street, someone had shown him a love that passes all understanding (and of knowing the love of Christ that passes knowledge, so that you are filled to the measure of all the fullness of God. Ephesians 3:19) and it is the love of God demonstrated through the sacrifice of his son Jesus Christ on the cross, who had transformed his life and could do it for others as well.

I listened to this music and it really touched my heart, it was as if I was listening to God calling me, to Jesus Christ, to this immense love, what I heard in the church I was listening to now on the radio.

It was so great that I wanted to be part of it, I wanted to get closer to God so I went back to church and received Jesus as the Lord and Savior of my life it was something totally beautiful really my life began to change everything was wonderful, my Life that was normally quiet began to be extraordinary when I gave my heart to Jesus Christ.

Everything started to go much better, so to speak, I was going through a peak and very happy in my life, although I had grown up in a Christian family, since my parents' divorce when I was a teenager, I had moved away from the church and worse still I had stopped talking to God, but now that I had returned to God I was complete, physically, spiritually content, I had already acquired my university degree, I felt fulfilled, I could practically say that I was not missing anything at that stage of my life very grateful and happy.

Chapter Three: A calm day

I was on a normal day, a sparkling sun began, the song of the birds was happily heard as every morning they came to the tree that was located in the middle of my backyard. Everything seemed to be going normally. The usual gym workout routine, once I finished my university studies, I no longer had to go to college, but I was still preparing my documents to start looking for a job with my new and recently acquired university degree.

I was visiting the church regularly during the afternoon services, and I was very happy about everything that was happening in my life back then, until I started to feel a slight symptom out of the normal in my body. I thought it was something unimportant like a headache to which you take a pill and then it goes away a few hours later; Or maybe I thought, "I just need to lie down a bit and everything will pass." A nap will be the best so I decided it was a simple thing. I looked for a tablet in the pharmacy and I took it, I thought that everything would be fine in a moment, but, as perhaps you are thinking, after the moment things did not go well.

One day passed, then the next and the symptom, although it was almost imperceptible continued and I thought that perhaps I should comment it with some friendship that a small ailment like this had happened to him, I imagined that surely there would be another better tablet than the one I bought; I spoke on the phone with a family member and she told me her advice. He replied: Well, when I feel a little pain I take this one, perhaps the one you took was not as effective. Thinking about this I went to the pharmacy I bought a different tablet, from another laboratory, although with the same effect. As you can imagine I rested, but the symptom persisted. That being the case, after about a week I decided to go to the doctor so that he would completely eliminate the symptom since for me it was something unimportant, but perhaps, deep down inside, there was a doubt in me about what might actually be happening.

Usually we like to be in control of the situation around us, we like to know what time is it? How long is the journey we will undertake? At what age should we do this or that, we want to know everything, and be in control of everything, so that when something is out of our control we feel suspicious, and more so when something threatens our daily routine to which we are accustomed.

We even get used to feeling the same temperature level, if the weather changes, we feel threatened, like wondering what is going on? Is it winter or summer time? We are very much in control of what is happening around, so I said: although it is a symptom practically without much pain or discomfort I will go to the doctor since I do not want to feel this symptom, I want everything to be the same as the rest of my days before starting to feel this; I will pass consultation to annihilate this symptom of my life.

I went to the doctor's office, I remember that someone was having a consultation, so the nurse told me to wait my turn.

Everything was so happy for me that I enjoyed the time outside the office, I took my cell phone, I played a little something on my cell phone for a while, then I checked pictures from the gallery, I read messages stored in the mailbox and all that until I heard my name mentioned, it was the turn of consultation, I kept the phone, I exposed the case to the doctor and he told me that I had to do some tests before I could know what was happening. I thought he would just tell me take an effective pill and the discomfort will come out, but I thought it was okay to do it his way, doctors always like to do things more elegantly and say things in a more scientific way, do so much business to finally tell me: you are fine, you can go.

That was my thought, so I said well, if it is necessary to do these tests so that he can finally say "he can go, everything is fine", I will. So I left there for the laboratory to do the corresponding exams.

I got there with one might say sarcastic laughter or maybe, I don't know, I thought it was all fun for me, being in the laboratory I did the required tests and they said: "Come back the next day for the result" which I spent one afternoon happy.

It never crossed my mind that I was going to go through more than just taking a tablet and everything would be fine, since I thought that way, I didn't care about it, I did the rest of my daily activities as usual and went home.

☐

Chapter four: The moment

The day came to withdraw the results of the medical examinations, I happily carried out my normal routine of each day; a healthy breakfast, exercise, watch regular tv shows and went to the lab to get the results. It was my enthusiasm to go look for them to show them to the doctor since I thought: "I just have to go and get the doctor's approval, go buy the required tablet that he indicates and everything will be fine.

With that expectation I withdrew the results of the laboratory, took the taxi and went to the doctor's office with the exams in hand, I waited for my turn again, they mentioned my name and I passed, it could be said with a kind of smile on my face. I was grateful to God for the new day he was giving me and I gave the tests to the doctor, he took them, began to review them and was silent.

I remember that I was distracted on my cell phone because he took a while to talk to me again, he asked me some questions about my health, which I answered positively well according to my diagnosis. I remember that I was distracted on my cell phone because he took A little while talking to me again, he asked me some questions about my health, which I answered positively well according to my diagnosis.

He asked me: Have you been healthy? do you exercise Have you had a disease in the past that required surgery? to which I said no.

In my table of diagnostic questions (inside my mind) I had 100% approval for the rating of a healthy person.

The doctor continued to remain silent and review the exams, I became distracted again seeing anything on my phone when then he spoke again, he told me that he had something to say to me but that he needed me to be mature and serene enough to listen to him; he said to me: "sit well", this is something you need to take it easy.

When I listened to that introduction, before giving me a result, all my insides told me that something was not right because the doctor's face had changed, there seemed to be a certain regret in his eyes, which did not indicate a good sign since who asked me to remain calm before listening to what he had to say to me.

In a quiet, almost comforting voice, he asked me once more to stay calm, I don't know how to explain it, but, immediately that request activated my heart one hundred percent and what accelerated was heart palpitations so strong and so fast that I felt that it could come out of my chest, inside I said:

"Say what you are going to say!"

I could no longer bear such anguish, now I do not know what will happen to me, I began to get so nervous that I did not care about the cell phone anymore, I did not care about anything else that was around me, I just wanted to know what he had to say to me. doctor.

I was silent and then I told him that I was ready to listen to him, so he began to explain to me why I shouldn't feel bad when listening to what he would tell me, had the examinations revealed that I was going through a - "terminal stage disease" - he asked me since when did I have symptoms of this? - I told him that at the most one week a slight symptom started and I thought that it was the same as the headache that one takes any pill and then it only becomes a bad memory.

He asked me if I had not had ailments and strong symptoms months ago, I said no, then he bowed his head and looked at me with more regret than before and said: Then we are facing an unusual case, as we say popularly one by one. million, very rarely this disease develops silently in the patient without giving any symptoms in his body; That is your case, he told me, you are in the terminal stage of this disease and although I do not want to tell you in this way:
"There is no medical procedure that can help you, there is nothing we can do because of the advanced stage of the disease."

I felt as if the world had literally fallen onto my back, leaving my body crushed in that office chair, because it is one thing to be told you have this disease, and although it is not the best news in the world, but, when this news comes accompanied by the following word of encouragement: "But with this treatment we are going to face it until you come out of this and you are better" - that gives you encouragement, in my case it was not.

I was told you have this and there is no hope because you are in a terminal stage, there is no process that we try to help you due to the advanced stage of the disease, so it was as if the news was already accompanied by the farewell ticket, as when they tell you Game Over in a video game and your life time is up; I mean, I didn't have time to try to do something to remedy things. So I said to him: But how so? what can we do? What can I take of medicine?

I thought he was going to tell me to take this medicine and everything will be fine, he answered no, he told me: - The disease developed silently in your body and now you have this small and slight symptom that is indicating that the stage is ending and it only remains little time to live, I do not want to say it, but it is the end of the cycle so, he said, we could carry out exams to try to help you but I tell you once the possibilities are practically nil, possibly you are going to undergo the procedures without any results.

The diagnosis is: There is nothing more to do, but if you want to undergo processes it will be at your risk because I do not assure you of any possibility. I was then silent and he said to me: Well, here are your papers, I have to continue attending; It's your decision.

I took the results of my exams and I got out of there I do not even know how, I felt that everything was spinning around, I remember that it was midday and although the sun was sparkling as the one that brightened my mornings, at that moment I felt as if everything was gray, millions passed of thoughts through my head and I couldn't find a coherent idea, an idea with meaning in me.

I remember that I left the door of the clinic, there were people on the street, cars and I stayed on the outside wall, I could not get an idea, if I took a taxi to go home or stay in the park and take a little of air; I wasn't sure what I would do with my life from that moment on, but there was a light deep inside me, since a short time ago I had given my life to Christ.

I understood that he had died on the cross for love and I thought that love was so great, what was he who I wanted to be with at that moment, so, I raised my eyes to heaven and said I am in your hands my Lord, that immediately brought To my strength, knowing that this great love was with me brought me calm and peace in the midst of the terrible storm I was going through, so I could breathe, I stopped a taxi and went home.

Chapter five: In the middle of the storm

When I got home being in my room I let out the tears, I cried and cried, the tears came out without any effort, I cried so much that my eyes were already well swollen and I felt that I needed to vent all the uncertainty that was enclosing inside me. I thought within myself: I will no longer be able to develop the career for which I studied for five years at university, I will no longer have children or start a family like every young woman expects, there were no dreams to achieve, the daily routine that I carried out nothing mattered anymore and there was no reason to be, because death stalked my life in an imminent way.

Facing this reality I poured out my life and my heart in tears, but in his great mercy God knocked on the door of my heart and reminded me that even in this time without exit he was there, his love was not exhausted; Then I remembered Job's life in the Bible when he lost everything, his possessions, his family, even his health and he said: Jehovah gave Jehovah took away, may Jehovah's name be blessed. (Job 1: 21-22)

This reminded me that everything comes from God, all the good things we have, all the blessings, each day we live is a gift and many times we do not value it.

Every time we open our eyes and we can see the sparkling sun that shines on everyone, we do not give it the importance and gratitude it deserves, just because we do not have brand name shoes that appear on the cell phone screen, or because we could not download the fashionable song and we forget that around us there are enormous gifts that God gives us every day, and they go unnoticed because our interests take us away from what is really important in this life, God, life, our loved ones.

So it was with me and I, faced with this reality that I was going through, said: "Thank you God", with my eyes full of tears, "Thank you God", up to here you have allowed me to live, you have allowed me to see each sunrise; Every day you have given me beautiful moments, health, I was the one who did not know how to value all the time what was in front of me, and now that I was facing the possibility of never having them again, then I realized how much they mattered, but , it was late.

However, I continued saying "Thank you God", I do not understand what happened and it hurts, but still above my emotions, "Thank you God" because you have loved me since before the foundation of the world, (as he chose us in it before the foundation of the world, that we might be holy and blameless before him. Ephesians 1: 4), you have been faithful thanks, praying this the tears dried in my eyes and I could rest a little in my bed.□

Chapter six: The search begins

A new day dawned, I prayed to God, I thanked him because he was still alive. I was ready inside to go out looking for new options. I thought that maybe the doctor could have been too drastic in his diagnosis and a second medical opinion could give me hope, a treatment to follow.

Thinking about it I even went to another city, I started the journey in search of new answers, I prayed and I said to the Lord: I know that you have the power to change this diagnosis or give me an exit, a treatment, I will travel to this city and I hope hear something new. With that hope I started the bus trip of about three and a half hours, I was so focused on the goal that I couldn't even feel the time of the trip. I felt like I had entered the bus and then got off immediately.

My mind did not want to think about anything other than a new diagnosis, so I came to the other city, took the taxi to the clinic and when I had a consultation, I found a doctor, I thought:

Wow, things are getting better!

As a woman, just like me, perhaps she can empathize with me and look for answers, not like the other doctor who, according to me, was very bad (I think that in my despair, my mind was looking for something to hold on to), so I entered excited, with hopes , I explained what had happened and the diagnosis I had received, she told me: "I need to see your exams" - I gave them to her right away, she kept looking at me and said: the doctor was right, that is her condition, she is in terminal stage and where do you come from? - I wonder. I told him that I had traveled from another city, he told me: You should not have done it in your terminal stage condition, you must be at home and wait for the moment, when I heard this, all the positivism I was carrying fell to the ground, I think my face reflected my I am disconsolate because she, upon seeing my reaction, added: if you want, we can do procedures, but I warn you that they will be painful and the chances that they will be null.

Do you really want to submit to them? If you do it it will be at your risk, in a terminal stage it is very difficult to see a positive result, but, if you want to do it, the decision is in your hands. I thought it was a good idea to do it, even if I had no chance of success, but I thought that if that was the way God was going to help me, however small that possibility might be, I could be free of all that I was experiencing.

I told her that I was willing to undergo whatever procedures were necessary, however painful they were. That being the case, he gave me an appointment for a time, meanwhile he prescribed medicine for me to take effect before the day of the medical intervention. Having said that, I went straight from there to a pharmacy to buy the medicine, it was expensive by the way and the application quite uncomfortable so it was a difficult time but I did not mind, I was hopeful about the possibility of improving my health through all that.

I did everything as instructed, and looking forward to the day when the medical intervention would take place, I placed my trust in God. While waiting for the date of the appointment I thanked God every day, although, to be honest, it was difficult for me to smile just like before when I knew how little life time I had left. ☐

Chapter seven: Facing pain

The day of the long-awaited medical intervention has arrived and really went beyond what I thought. I had taken the medicine as it had been indicated and that filled me with high hopes, the day came without knowing what to expect.

Once I was in front of the doctor she told me: Take off your clothes, put on your robe and let's start. They prepared everything on site and we started; He explained that this was a procedure in which he could not use anesthesia, so he asked me to please not move. Feel what you feel you cannot move –he exclaimed- we are going to try to cauterize the entire area, we are going to use a laser to burn hoping to cauterize the entire affected area and thus be free of the affection that your body faces.

I agreed, I thought within myself: Although this is not the best intervention I expected to receive, but it is the only way left, let's do it, so he started that extremely painful intervention, it lasted a short time and then he told me: You are ready!

Leave the body lying down for a while, regain strength, take a breath and then get dressed and go home. Although I had felt pain without anesthesia I could breathe an air of positivity as I thought, I have waited for a long time for this moment, I followed the required instructions and now I am in this phase without any problem.

Meditating this made me very happy, I took a breath, got dressed and then went to his office; There she explained that everything had gone well, the process went well, but she told me: Everything is hurt now, it is not possible to detect if the intervention was successful or not, so we are going to wait two weeks until we can see with certainty if we were successful.

It was time to go home, so I took that transport to my city and I only had to wait the waiting time. During my recovery I would go to church, sing to God songs of praise, of gratitude, sing with my heart and say to him I am in your hands, I trust you, so as time went by I tried to follow my life with a rhythm similar to normal I had before.

However, although I could eat and walk and aesthetically I saw the same thing, I carried out my usual routine of life, deep down there was regret for the health situation I was going through, although I could recognize that only thank God that health process did not I managed to collapse completely, I could feel that God was with me to advance each day expecting the uncertain since nothing was safe in that daily life.
☐

Chapter eight: During the wait

I remember that in those times there was a beautiful activity in the church where I attended. They invited preachers from another country to share time together on the word of God.

Despite my health circumstances, I always tried to be close to God, every time there was service in the church, I tried to attend and this beautiful activity was no exception. I must admit that I was not completely excited to go since it was not easy for me to smile happily in the middle of what I was going through, but in the same way, God gave me the strength and I was able to enlist in the middle of my situation and I left with my heart willing to listen to the word of God.

The time of praise began and the way of listening to how God loves us through the musical melody was very beautiful. Everything was beautiful around me, then the person in charge of giving the teaching came to the altar and said: - The Lord has told me that there are three women here, who at this time have diagnosed serious illnesses, I want to pray for them, now come on up front, you know who you are. I did not know who the others were, but I knew that I had been diagnosed with something very difficult so I decided to go forward, while I was crossing the place I saw two more women approaching, there were three of us in total as he had said, so he he extended his hands and prayed for us, I don't remember exactly what he said, but I do remember the end of the prayer, the brother said: "They are healthy" the Lord heals them.

It was a special moment for me because I heard the phrase: "The Lord says heal her" so I received that word deep in my heart and cried with gratitude, I was so grateful to God because not only had He loved me and had been with me from the beginning of this circumstance, but now he told me that I was healthy.

At the end of the service we returned to our places, I was very happy. So much was my contentment that time passed and it was time to travel again to pass the medical consultation where I would finally know if the intervention had been successful or not.

I was going with a different expectation, I had already received in the church the word that said "the Lord heals her", very happy and much more positive than before, I took the bus, traveled to the office and arrived with very high standards of positive expectation , so I went in and the doctor sent me to change, put on my robe to check myself, inside I was really very happy and said to myself: My ears will enjoy hearing the doctor say - you are totally healthy - yes I imagined the way I would hear that.

The checkup ended, I left the dressing room and to my surprise after the doctor checked me there was no comment, I even went back to sit in front of the doctor, but I did not hear that the phrase I expected was spoken by the doctor's lips.

When the period of silence began to extend I thought: I think something is wrong and, confirming my suspicions, the doctor told me: "Her condition has worsened", the intervention we did was not successful, the disease is progressing much more. Humanly I felt myself collapse, it was not what I wanted to hear, it was not the best thing I could hear at this moment in my life because I had the desire to live, to achieve my goals and dreams, but now I was faced with the fact that the disease had advanced a lot more and that the medical intervention had not had any results.

The frustration was evident on my face, so the doctor told me: I warned you that we could intervene but that there were practically no possibilities because you are in the terminal stage, I thanked him for his time and I left there with my documents in hand and also with my feelings shattered.

I went to take the bus back home and despite my circumstance I did not dare to claim God asking why, I simply said to him: I do not understand the process but I always trust you my God, you said that we were healed but I did not understand if it really was healed in my heart, if it was the soul that was being healed to be able to leave in peace or if it was the body and I said I don't understand the process and I don't understand what happened but I still trust you my God, this prayer gave me rest and I was able to finish getting home.

When I arrived I began to pray thanking God for everything, even if I did not understand it, then I closed the possibility of continuing to travel to this office because there was nothing else to do it for.
☐

Chapter nine: Aimlessly

A stage of uncertainty began to haunt my mind, having already seen two medical opinions from different places, the diagnosis remained the same, you are in the terminal stage and there is nothing we can do for you.

It was then in my despair, I was aimless, trying to find answers, I thought that perhaps the doctors in my country were not as specialized as the doctors in more developed countries (due to the limited scientific and technological resources of my country), I thought that perhaps there would be an answer in another place outside the country because he had already gone to one city and another and had not found an answer.

I figured that maybe the training that doctors in more developed countries have could help me, I had this thought in mind when I talked on the street with someone who told me about a place that was receiving medical help from other countries, that just in the week that We were, a brigade of doctors from the United States had arrived in the country, with technological equipment that they brought from there, and although I had not told him anything about my health, this comment came out in conversation spontaneously, the person also added: Someone I know went to spend consultation with the North American doctors and he says they have very advanced medical equipment and they even gave this person the medicine.

Immediately I felt as if a light of hope lit up again in me and I thought: I have a new opportunity so I asked the exact address and what hours they were attending so I could attend. Without waiting, I went home, changed and got my papers ready; I went to that place hoping to find no obstacles along the way since I had the firm conviction that there was the answer I had been waiting for.

I arrived at the place and I didn't even have to wait, immediately I was going to be attended, there was an American doctor attending, she spoke English and little Spanish, but I had studied English in the time I was going to university and given this, I quite understood what she was saying the doctor.

He told me to change, I will check you, he said. I went to change with a joy that I could not hide, then I showed her the exams, the doctor told me: Lie down on the table, which I did immediately, she checked me out. Then, I changed, I sat down and once again I was waiting to hear the phrase "you are healthy" or "you have this treatment option to return to have your health restored", I was already beginning to despair to hear this phrase at which the doctor said: This disease has progressed aggressively and you are in a terminal condition, there is nothing that medicine can do for you.

At that time, she explained to me that no matter how advanced the studies are, it does not depend on the progress of the studies but on the stage of the disease, medical advances allow us to help patients to get out of this. when the disease is detected in its earliest stages.

That was the complete opposite of what I had expected to hear. I got out of there, I'm not sure if more lost and devastated than before.
It was very hard for me.

☐

Chapter ten: Attached to life

It was already the third medical opinion in my case, which left me with very little chance of finding a different diagnosis. In my city the first medical opinion was frustrating for me, I received the exact same diagnosis in another city, I came back and taking advantage of the fact that there was a brigade of North American doctors with advanced technology in the country, I visited them and to my surprise or greater frustration the diagnosis was the same.

Despite me, the circumstance, there was a living hope in me, I do not understand how but I still expected to hear at some point: "The situation has a solution", I hoped to hear at some point that everything would be better, that I should only follow some medicine new or some kind of way my circumstance might be different.
While my real options were running out, I was subject to faith in God, I trusted that he was in control of everything, even when I did not understand it, there was a living hope that did not let my faith fall apart.

Being this way I was in my usual city, my usual routine, although now with the disease in tow.
I decided to try once again to do something to change my situation, I heard about a modern clinic in my city with advanced technology and specialized doctors.

So many good references I heard, I thought that it could be an option to end this process that was happening, that I would find a place where they would not repeat to me that things were getting worse and that there is nothing to do.

Despite the previous failures and disappointments, I decided to try one more time. I went to the place mentioned and to add more difficulty to my life than I already had with me, I realized that this place was really expensive, the consultation very high compared to the places I had visited before, they indicated that, to be attended there , I had to do the medical exams in their laboratory again, and as expected, each one had a high price.

Although I had already spent a lot of money on previous consultations and trips, I decided to try it again, I had practically no money left, I considered the possibility of getting the money borrowed or requesting help, I was not sure what I would do, but, my instinct human, the desire to survive, I clung to life, to fight until the last moment, so this is what I did once again.
☐

Chapter eleven: Face to face

I found the clinic with state-of-the-art technological advances and immediately I went to consult to expose my situation. Actually, the fame that place had was meritorious, everything there was very sharp and technologically advanced, different from the places I had visited before, that gave me an air of joy.

I entered the office that was indicated to me, I carried out the required exams and then the doctor saw my results, listened to my version and told me: Let's review it, a spark of hope ignited in me, I longed to hear the words: "You are healthy", "God has made a miracle in your life" - because every night I cried and asked God to help me in this situation.

Thinking about this I lay down on the stretcher and once checked, I was waiting for the phrase I wanted to hear.

After getting dressed I came to talk to the doctor, she explained that we could do a more detailed analysis to see how deep the involvement was in my body and what mechanisms to follow, if there was a possibility, I told her that it was fine. I wanted to know everything, I was prepared to listen to whatever was necessary because I had no other choice. The doctor had a machine similar to the one that ultrasounds do to moms when they go to see their baby, I think it was the same machine, I'm not sure, but well, there was a screen where I could see my interior myself, so she put a sort of gel on my body and then the machine part started to pass by and I could observe my body.

I looked away from the screen for a moment and I think I just hoped to hear that there was no condition in my body and I was healthy. The doctor told me: Look at the screen and see - this is your body and this is the condition it is in. For the first time I could see the damage that was inside me and I could see face to face the disease that had been attacking me and ending my health all this time.

The doctor toured my body and told me this is the affected area, so far it has reached, this is the place that leads to other organs and more, so that is the reason why you cannot put anesthesia in the procedures, because It is located very close to delicate organs and it is very dangerous for you to be unconscious since you will not be able to have any reaction during surgery, if you go to another organ or something like that the damage would be irreparable.

In my understanding that was the matter, of course she told me in more sophisticated terms, you will understand that doctors speak in terms that sometimes do not seem to be in the same human language that one speaks, but, from what I could understand, that was the idea of what he was saying to me.

He told me that there was only one procedure left to do, he explained that it consisted of cutting all that area shown on the screen and removing it, this with the hope that the disease was lodged in this first layer of skin and he told me that many patients when removing them the first layer of skin is free of the disease since the second layer of skin is healthy and they only heal at the right time and survive.

This seemed great to me, but it also explained to me the other risk involved in this surgery. In the worst case, it may happen that after removing the first layer of skin and the disease has progressed to a second and third, nothing could be done.

I felt it was a risk that I should take. The cost of this intervention was very high and was beyond my capacity. With difficulty I had been able to adjust to do the analysis to which I was subjected and performing the intervention was not within my financial reach.

My face seemed unable to hide my anguish when needing the intervention, but not having enough money to do it.

While trying to find a possible solution in my head, the doctor gave me the photographs of my situation, which she had seen on screen, and apparently she noticed the sadness on my face since it was difficult for me to get that amount, so she said: I have had patients who face this procedure and do not have the money to pay for it, so they go to the local public hospital, they also carry out this intervention, what I can do is give you an order indicating the process you need to carry out and Hopefully, doing so will give you a positive and satisfactory result. I expressed to her that I would have liked her to intervene in that surgery, but I did not have the money to pay for it, so I accepted the order to go to the public hospital.
☐

Chapter twelve: The last wagon

I attended the public place indicated by the doctor, I presented my case once again, I explained the history of what had been happening and they told me: In your case, you no longer have a reliable cure, it is in a terminal stage and there is nothing we can do for you, we are caring for people who have life chances, we cannot stop caring for someone who will live to care for you, we cannot have a stretcher busy with someone who in any case has to leave, we cannot offer any type of service given its terminal condition, what we can do is recommend that you go home to wait for the moment.

Although I knew my condition, that was the last thing I wanted to hear, so my eyes filled with tears and I could not find a way to answer, the words were hidden from my mouth, but as I could I said: "Please, there must be somehow, I'm young and I want to live", please I exclaimed in a pleading voice. When listening to me, the person who treated me told me: There is a medical extension here from the hospital, which helps cases of women. I can give you the information there if you want; You have two options, you can go home or you can try going to that place to see what they can do for you. I thanked him for the information and his time serving me.

I left there with this last hope and I said inside: It seems that the time has come, I looked for options, I fought, I tried and apparently this is the last train car, I can't find an answer, it will be all.

At the same time that I left the hospital, I went to that place that they indicated and how I thought it was a kind of consultation or something, I did not warn at home that I would go to see this other option, I assumed that we would talk and then we would analyze the options to do so I came to the place, according to me, I was just going to ask what would happen, if there would be possibilities of doing something or not.

To my amazement when I arrived, they analyzed my case and told me: Are you aware that you have a terminal illness, that there is no chance of success in the intervention we carry out? I said yes, they have told me many times - I added.

The doctor who was treating me asked me if, even with that diagnosis, I wanted to try, she explained that the intervention was very painful since they could not apply anesthesia, she is aware of this - she told me. We have to cut without anesthesia on your body in a delicate area and you will have to bear all that.

Conscious of it I said to him: yes we do it. I thought he would schedule me the appointment to perform the procedure, but without asking anything else, he began to give orders to the medical team that was there, bring oxygen, bring everything, prepare the area - said the doctor.

I wasn't sure what was happening and I asked her: When are you going to do the surgery? He replied - "right now".

At that moment I thought about making a call home, but she said in a loud voice: I turned off her cell phone immediately, it is no longer time to be on her cell phone, she should have called before coming here. That being the case, I did not have time to tell anyone anything and I thought to myself: I was looking for answers and the answer was here. I was a little satisfied with that thought and I decided to follow the indicated procedure.

While I was waiting, I watched as they were preparing all the necessary medical tools before my eyes, then I thought about God, I remembered that in the Bible God says: I will never leave you, I will never abandon you, do not fear because I am your God who strives you, who holds you by your right hand and says do not fear, I help you. (Because I, Jehovah, am your God, who holds you by your right hand, and says to you: Fear not, I will help you. Isaiah 41:13) then I could feel a peace within me when I remembered this passage from the Bible, this promise from God and I literally felt like someone stood next to the head of the bed when it all started.

I could not move due to the doctor's indication, due to the delicacy of the surgery. I remember that person or character who was standing there gave me so much peace and so much confidence in the process. Since it all started, the nurses were there around me and the pain started, when I agreed to perform the surgery without anesthesia, I completely ignored the magnitude of the suffering I was going to experience. I could feel every part of me being cut, I couldn't even cry from the pain because this would make my body shake or sway and I should not make the slightest movement.

In the middle of that scene that seemed like terror, I remember that I took with my hand the metal railing of the stretcher I was on and I remember that I felt it as if it were a plasticine bar, the exaggerated pain I was experiencing made me perceive the sensation as if the metal railing bent in my hand; I think he was delirious from the pain, but then, I could feel the presence of that character by my side during the process and he transmitted calm to me, I thought: that nurse who stood there next to the head of my bed, surely she is Christian and He surely prays a lot because since he stopped there I have felt a lot of peace, maybe God sent her to remember him and think about him, his promises and everything he had read in the Bible about his fidelity, about his love and on how he always tried to be there for his people in the worst difficulties.

The process finally ended and everyone started to leave the room, the doctor said that everything had gone well and recommended that I stay resting for a moment, because due to the injuries she should not move, we are going to wait a few minutes so she can put on her clothes.

Everyone left the room except the character who was next to the head of my bed, I wanted to turn around to thank him for his company, I wanted to ask him his name or know him, but when I turned my head gently there was no one there, at least not someone visible Humanly, it was then when I understood that who had been by my side was God, I could not see him with my natural eyes but if I felt it all the time, he did not leave me alone for a moment as he promised in his word, he was with me just as it is in our lives when we need it but many times our occupations prevent us from feeling it, generally we are too busy to be able to feel his presence, many times we are so stressed as to be able to feel his love taking care of us, waiting for us.

So I prayed and thanked God because he had survived that process, because he had been with me and had helped me to be successful.
☐

Chapter thirteen: The final result

After the intervention, he had to wait eight days to be able to go in search of the long-awaited final result. I did not feel the days of so much craving that I had to know the answer.

When the moment finally came, she was happy, thanking God that she could breathe, because she was alive, and because she was almost certain that the result would finally be the healing she so longed for.

I went to the place and very happy I waited for my turn to pass the consultation. When I arrived with the doctor, she treated me with a cold look, without any expression on her face, she mentioned my name and I said yes, it is me, she said - the result of the intervention is here, but even so, I need to check you. He checked me, then he said: Put your clothes back on, I need to talk to you.

I expected to jump with joy when hearing news of healing, but I waited for her to mention it, the doctor looked me straight in the eye and said: The disease progressed.

Then she began to explain to me, she said: We removed the infected part in the first layer of her body, but the disease is in the other layer and we can no longer remove any more parts because then we would have to cut you to pieces, that would be the same as killing you so there is nothing more to do, we cannot continue damaging your body because the disease has already advanced beyond what humanly we could have remedied.

He prescribed me a huge list of medicines and told me: Take it daily for the rest of the time, try to be calm, if you are anxious the pain will increase and you will not be able to bear it then, take the medicine and it will help to calm the pain.

I asked her how much time I had left, she told me about three months to live. That remains if you sleep as necessary, take care of yourself and lead a normal rhythm of life, if you do not despair, you can reach three months otherwise the time will shorten.

This is an estimate based on how the disease has been reacting, but I cannot tell you exactly how much.

This news for me was devastating, although from the beginning they told me that he was in the terminal phase, I did not think that he would last so little time with life.

Stunned by the fatal news, I took my documents, thanked the doctor for her time and patience. I was devastated, my feelings and my hopes had reached the end of the road, I had neither the strength nor the desire to try anything else; I was sore both physically but also in my soul.

I looked at the sky and said to the Lord: I am in your hands, if you want you can take me right now and not wait three months, I am in your hands Lord. It seemed as if God was silent and just watching me.

I walked to a nearby pharmacy and asked how much the medicine I was supposed to take daily would cost, the cost for the medicine was extremely high and I couldn't even buy the dose for one day, the price of the dose for one day was about $ Approximately $ 60.00, at that time that amount was almost equal to the cost of a month's salary for an average worker in my country, I had no money for a day's dose of medicine and less to take it daily for three months, so no I bought the entire prescription, I think I bought a pill to try to follow the doctor's instructions, but after I had bought it I thought: why do I buy one? - I must buy the whole dose but I do not adjust with the money, then I thought: Even if I adjusted to buy it, why do it if it will not cure me anyway, it is only to wait for the time of my departure.

So I said to myself: I won't spend what little money I have left on a medicine that won't heal me anyway.

I decided to keep what little money I had, I went home and once again I cried without consolation because there was no more hope.

I entered my room, I prayed to the Lord and I said to him: God of my life, you know that I love you and although this process that I do not understand is happening, I still trust you, God here is my life, the doctors say they are missing a few months for me to leave this land, if you want to take me you can take me now, I'm ready, or you can take me whenever you want but, if you want you can heal me, I promise that if you heal me, for the rest of my life I will tell you what that you did in me, I remember that I had cried as much as I could and I raised this prayer with all my heart, with all my soul, with all my mind and with all that I had of strength then I fell asleep until the next day.
☐

Chapter fourteen: Speechless

Time began to pass, I remember that the first week after that final result counted the days. I said to myself: Three days less, four days less, five days and so on. After a while, I stopped counting and thought: God you are with me, no matter what day it is or when the time comes, I am ready and I want to live for you the time I have left. I felt as if God had given me the strength to stop worrying, to get up in the midst of that health situation that was distressing my soul.

Due to my limited financial budget I had not bought medical treatment and I decided to trust only God, I began to live what I had left of life in a normal way, I went to church and sang with such joy that nobody could suspect what I was going on.

I was determined to live for God the time I was on this earth; I was able to share many moments of joy in the church as time passed.

I remember someone telling me that they were looking for staff in a new pharmacy that would open in the city, I had run out of options professionally due to the disease, although I had already finished university, I had not continued trying to advance my professional life.

So I thought maybe it wasn't a bad idea to give myself a chance to have a new experience, work and live fully before the day came.

I decided to go to spend the job interview, to my amazement, they gave me the position and I started working there. I really knew many nice people and whenever I could I told them about God, about how beautiful it is to have God in our lives who never abandons us, even in the worst moments.

We developed a very nice work environment, I got along very well with my coworkers and I remember that the pharmaceutical laboratories always came to train us, explain us about the properties of the products and how to help patients who came in search of medications.

While both laboratories arrived, I remember that almost a year had passed since that consultation where I received the final result of my health condition, and it was then that someone came to offer a free examination on the type of illness I had in my body. This seemed strange to me since it is not very common that exams are offered like this, they are only done to people who are going through this type of situation and he offered a co-worker and me this exam.

I meditated for a moment and then I questioned why a year had passed since my last result and I was still alive, I remembered that it was only three months that I was supposed to live, I looked at the sky and inside

I said to the Lord: Is this part of your plan? - I did not receive any response from God.

So I rejected the exam and said: No, I do not want to know about medicines or something like that, I had arranged in my heart not to try any more medical interventions or treatments, I had arranged that the day it was time to leave, because I would go and ready but I decided I would not undergo medical treatment again.

My co-worker insisted and said to me: Go do it, anyway, you don't have that disease; I remembered that she did not know what I had been through, I had not told anyone about my work. So I decided to take that test and I said to God: If this is part of your plan, that's fine, it will be as you want. So I took it and the next week as prescribed in the invitation I went to take the exam.

This time everything was different, I had been in consultation before and I no longer expected to hear anything positive because I was aware of my situation, I had only attended because I trusted God and I thought: I do not know what he has prepared for me, but I was not going with some expectation as before where I was wanting to dominate every situation, always anticipating what I would hear.

This time I was trusting in what God wanted me to hear, and I had my whole life trusting in him, that's how the doctor reviewed me and asked: Why are you here? I meditated inside myself and thought: How strange that he did not tell me - the situation is worse and the same phrase as always that the doctors told me, so I replied: Well, doctor, I am here because they came to offer this exam and I also expressed all my case with the disease, I showed him the exams and he said: "Here is an error".

These medical tests have your name but they do not agree with what I have just reviewed at this moment, your body does not present what these papers say, I said to him: I am not understanding what doctor is saying, please explain, he replied: "You should not have this test because you are healthy", this test is for people who have this disease that these papers say, surely they are not yours and someone changed your clinical record; Your body is totally healthy, he told me, I did not know how to react to that response, I did not expect to hear something like that, I no longer expected to hear anything positive in my health, I even insisted saying to him, but I am in this condition and he replied: I say you have nothing, something annoying at my insistence asked me: Who is the doctor here, you or me? I replied: You are the doctor, so I tell you that you have nothing.

I just reviewed you, according to these medical papers, it says here that you had a last intervention, but you do not have a scar from any surgery, or any sign of previous treatment, it is as if these papers were not yours, if they were, you should have scars from the surgeries mentioned here, but you don't have them, you are totally healthy.

In the face of my notorious bewilderment, he took a sample from me and said: I see that you don't believe what I am saying, I will give you an order to repeat this test in a month, I will be on vacation, another doctor will have to attend.
I was speechless, before my silence the doctor added: I see that you do not believe what I say so go with this order, I need to attend more patients. I smiled and left immediately. I couldn't even put the thoughts in my mind, I sat down for a moment and I could only say: thank you God, thank you God because I am alive, because your love is so great and inexplicable, you are faithful and you are always in control.

At the indicated time, I returned to the office and a doctor attended me just as he had told me, she said to me: The doctor who treated you is on vacation. Everything was going as planned, then I heard that he said to me in a sharp voice: You should not come to this place to be late, we have serious patients to attend to, and you who have nothing come here, "this is not a joke, young lady".

I said to him: It is not a joke, it is that I have this medical file, but the doctor who treated me last time told me that this file did not show my health condition, he told me that I had nothing. Then she replied: If he told you that you have nothing, it is because it is so, in the analysis that was repeated before you consulted me today, it turns out that you are completely healthy, as indicated by the analysis you did and that The doctor who is on vacation reviewed you, I tell you that your body is like that of a girl who has never had any type of surgery, intervention or anything. "You are healthy" go to your house, I have patients to attend.

I thanked the doctor for her time, I did not mind that she was a little hostile to me, I was so happy that I could not contain so much joy. It was then that I understood that God had performed the miracle, I was completely healthy.

I did not take the medicine for a day, I had no hope, only Christ who shed his blood on Calvary's cross for love of us could give me freedom from that disease because his word says: by his wound we were healed, (He certainly took our illnesses, and he suffered our pains, and we considered him scourged, wounded by God and dejected, but he was wounded by our rebellions, crushed by our sins, the punishment of our peace was upon him, and by his stripes we were healed. Isaiah 53: 4-5).
That word is alive and Christ is still alive.

Christ died for love of us, but on the third day he rose with power and glory, and is seated at the right hand of God the Father.

Today Christ continues to heal, continues to perform miracles.

If you are sick or know someone who is suffering from some type of illness, tell them that Christ is still alive and that he continues to listen to the prayers of all who come to him from the heart.

Christ can do the miracle in your life how He did it with me.

CHRIST HEALED ME

CHRIST HEALED ME

CHRIST HEALED ME

He can heal you, and if you do not have a physical illness and you are sick in your soul, there are wounds that have marked and hurt you, Christ can also heal the wounds of the soul, of the heart in the human being.

When medicine has no answer for your physical condition, if you have been told that you can no longer heal because you are in the terminal stage of cancer, if you have still been diagnosed with AIDS, it does not matter what the disease is called or in the condition of advance that is, Christ is still alive and has power to heal, divine healing is real.

If you are reading this, it is because God also loves you and has a purpose for your life. He is waiting for you to approach him, to open the door of your heart to Christ and if you allow him to enter your heart he will never abandon you.
Christ loves you.

☐

Thanks

I thank God for the opportunity to write this book, and thus share the miracle of healing that he did in my life.

I am hopeful that through this testimony many people will know about the love and power of God.

Thanks to the sacrifice of Jesus Christ who shed his blood on Calvary's cross, today we can receive Salvation, but we can also receive healing, both physical and spiritual, and miracles of all kinds.

Christ lives and is always attentive to our prayers, do not hesitate.

Biographical data

Kenia Adit Acevedo Martínez, originally from Nicaragua, the fourth of five siblings; She grew up in an evangelical Christian setting. Presented to the Lord from the age of four months, she received a biblical formation during her growth that allowed her to know God from her childhood.

She studied at the university graduating as an Architect in graphic design with an emphasis in digital art, at the same time she studied the English language in a language center. Years later she graduated from the teaching career.

Currently, she is an active member of a local evangelical Christian church, where she continues to serve God, learning more and more from him and his inexhaustible love.